You Know You Have ADHD When...

By Julie Posey

To all of my friends and family blessed with ADD/ADHD

Preface

Recent studies reveal that an estimated 2.46 million children live with ADHD in the United States. Approximately 60% of these children do not outgrow ADHD and continue to cope with this disorder throughout adulthood. I was one of them.

There are many ways that one can find to cope with the symptoms of ADHD and how it manifests itself. Someone once said that humor was the best medicine and I believe that applies to many situations in life including most of my "ADD/ADHD moments."

In 2007 I began to keep a list of all of the things that I did that I later laughed about. When I told my friends and family about it, I began to hear about their "ADHD moments" too and I started keeping a log of those.

It it my hope that while others who have been blessed by ADD/ADHD read this book, they will know that they are not alone most of all, I would like to thank you for reading this book.

Julie Posey

Table of Contents

While Hanging Out at Home...

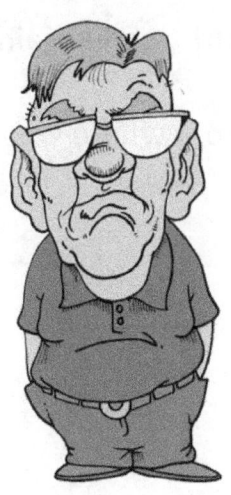

...you love the new vanilla scented body wash with moisture beads until you try to get the beads out of your hair.

...you've taken your coffee into the shower with you more than once.

...you have hidden a key to the house but when you are locked out, you can't find it to save your life.

...you clean and organize your house, but can't find anything that was there when you started.

...your home decorating scheme is "early American garage sale."

...you've had one wall left to paint in the living room for over two years.

...the cops have swarmed your home and ordered out with your hands above your head after you set off the burglar alarm and forgot your security code again.

...you lit a candle but can't remember where you sat it until one of the kids points out that your bed is on fire.

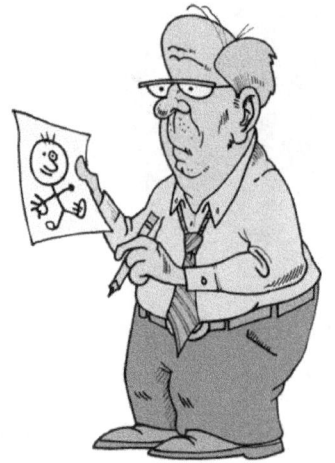

...you go to your mailbox to pick up today's mail and find the key is still in the lock from yesterday.

...the highlight of your day is to go to the mailbox so you can see all the things you ordered on eBay but forgot about.

...you have finally accepted that your house will never be neat and tidy but you still meet the pizza man at the curb for fear of embarrassment.

...you secretly pray that your mother will carry out her threat to toss your stuff in the trash if you don't clean up your room.

...you know that if a burglar ever entered your home, your state of disorganization would keep him from finding your valuables.

...you have to write a grocery list to remember less than five items.

...you go to the kitchen to warm up your coffee and realize you have no idea where your cup is for the third time this morning.

...you open the refrigerator and find the toothpaste you bought yesterday and the hairspray you lost a week ago.

...your cactus died because you forgot to water it.

...you go out to water the garden but end up spending the next hour washing the car.

...you've returned from the grocery store and suddenly remembered that before you left, you were filling the sink to wash dishes. Now, water has flooded the entire kitchen.

...you can find something in a pile of papers that doesn't appear to have any rhyme or reason to anyone but you.

...you walk in circles around the living room for hours searching for something and your spouse walks in and goes right to it.

...the front of your refrigerator is dedicated to all the sticky notes reminding you of all the things you need to do but you never look at those.

...you must have audible plant watering alarms or your plants would dry up and wilt away.

...your friends and family refer to your house as the plant hospice where plants come to die in dignity.

...you finally found the plant you bought last week at the farmer's market still in the trunk of your car.

...you can't grow plants even with an AeroGarden. You forget to look at the blinking lights to remind you to add water and nutrients.

...you forgot that you started some plants in the window sill between the window and storm window and they have thrived quite well but now you can't open the window without destroying them.

While Enjoying TV and Music...

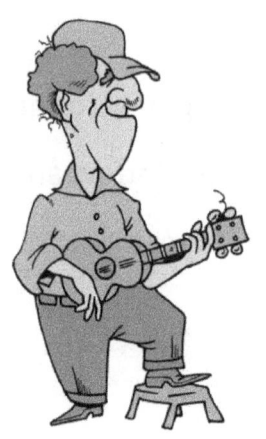

...you only have one album on your MP3 player and it takes you a week to realize it.

...you turn closed captioning on so that you can listen to your MP3 player and watch television at the same time.

...you've searched all day for your TV remote and finally find it in the refrigerator.

...your kids complain because you left the guide channel on the TV for more than five minutes.

...you have purchased at least three universal remotes for each television in the house.

...you spend 45 minutes trying to troubleshoot problems with the DVD player. Finally you realize that the reason your DVD won't play is because you keep putting the disc in the CD player.

...having the TV and stereo on at the same time actually helps you stay focused.

...you just can't watch a movie without getting up to go to the bathroom, going to get a snack, checking your e-mail or texting someone at least once every 15 minutes.

...your house has a power outage but you still you go to another room to watch TV.

...you wish you could record your daily activities and create an award winning reality show.

...you have to mentally sing the jingle for your favorite radio station so you can find it on the car stereo.

...your spouse pauses the movie every five minutes to stop and listen to every amazing and profound thing you have to say.

When ADD Involves Appointments or Events...

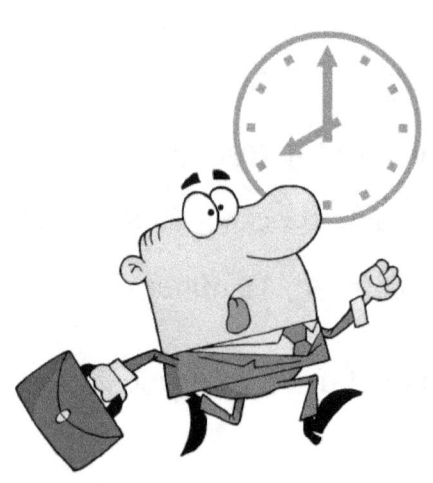

...you become mystified because you can't remember whether an event has already occurred or is about to occur.

...you must set an alarm to remind you to do something within the next 15 minutes.

...your friends point out that every calendar in your house is on a different month.

...for the third time this week you realize that you have double booked an appointment.

...you start to believe that you could simplify your life just by converting to Jehovah's Witness. Then you could eliminate holidays from your schedule.

...your friend sends you one of those book greeting cards and you've already become too distracted to read past the first page.

...you buy belated birthday cards a month before the birthday because you have already anticipated forgetting to mail them.

...you have to write a note to remember anything that occurred within the last 15 minutes.

...you are always at least 15 minutes late or 30 minutes early for everything.

...you have ever forgotten to attend a funeral and the family chose you as a pallbearer.

...the check your parents gave you for your birthday last year is still in your wallet.

...it isn't Halloween and you have real cobwebs covering your front door.

...you hide the Christmas presents you plan to give your kids and can't remember where they are on Christmas Eve.

...you buy your mother an exquisite pair of earrings with a matching necklace for her birthday in April, but she doesn't get them until Christmas.

...you buy birthday cards in pairs because you know you will lose one before you mail it.

...In February you notice that the Christmas cards from last year are still sitting on the coffee table. You put labels and stamps on them but never mailed them.

...your family considers it a holiday tradition after everyone has to evacuate your house when the all of the smoke alarms go off.

...you are over 30 and feeling guilty for never sending thank you notes to those who sent you high school graduation gifts.

...you are chosen as a potential juror in a highly publicized case but you can't remember the trip to the courthouse let alone what you've read in the newspaper about the case

While Using Computers or the Internet...

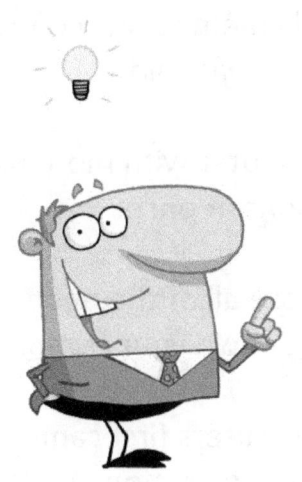

...you surf the Internet from your laptop on the couch so you can watch a movie at the same time.

...you decide that it is time to have the ink cartridges in the printer refilled. When you return home, your spouse informs you that the color one was almost full when you left.

...you install a browser with tabs so you can "power surf" in dozens of windows at once.

...you try to shew a fly off of your monitor screen by moving the mouse.

...you've used an instant messenger to ask a friend to call your cell phone so you can find it.

...you spend three hours looking for your WiFi password and your kids tell you the manufacturer put it on the bottom of the router for people like you.

...you save the e-mail messages you send so that you can review them to know what you said.

...you communicate with family members via e-mail so that you'll have a record of what was said.

...you had to upgrade your computer with more RAM so that you can open 70 applications at once.

...it takes you 15 minutes to close all of the open windows on your screen before shutting down your computer.

...you were intrigued when computers first came out. The speed at which they processed information and the ability to multitask was very impressive.

...your friends are puzzled by at least half of your Tweets and Facebook status updates.

...you are embarrassed by the number of times you've went to post a Facebook status update on a friend's wall.

...you mentioned something annoying about a friend in your latest Facebook status and then remembered he is on your friend list.

...you scratch your head trying to figure out how you know Tom from MySpace.

...you check in to places on Facebook just so you can remember where you've been.

...all of your friends know about the fight between you and your spouse because you clicked on forward instead of reply in the e-mail.

...your best friend posts on Facebook about the death of her grandmother and you click the "like" button.

...you are very embarassed when you post an inappropriate photo to your Facebook wall from your cell phone.

...you've put the wrong birthday in your Facebook profile and wonder why people are wishing you the happiest day ever.

While Cooking or Cleaning...

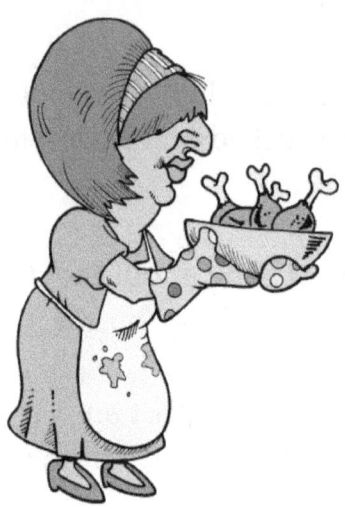

...you have lost at least one major part to each of your small kitchen appliances.

...you notice that you've just sprayed fabric freshener on your vegetables instead of vegetable cleaner.

...it takes you five minutes to figure out that no matter how long you press the can of beans against the coffee dispenser it is not the electric can opener and won't open your can.

...you know what month-old meat loaf looks like.

...caffeine helps you stay focused and calm.

...your husband turns on one of those shows about hoarders to scare you into cleaning the house.

...you live alone and still can't figure out who put the canned goods in the refrigerator.

...in the morning you expect to have coffee when you get out of the shower but realize you forgot to add coffee so there's a nice pot of hot water waiting for you.

...you notice that none of your family has finished their pumpkin pie. It might be because you forgot to add the sugar to the recipe.

...you have melted a hole in more than one teakettle.

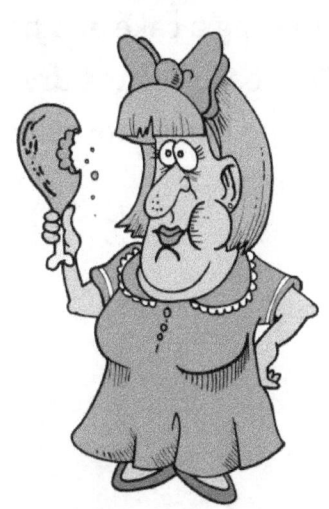

...you started buying glass mixing bowls after you melted all of the plastic ones sitting them on a hot burner.

...you leave part of the meal in the oven at least twice a week.

...you have attempted to cook potpies on the Foreman grill.

...you always double the recipe when making cookies so that you'll end up with a dozen that aren't burned.

...you spend all day preparing the food for Thanksgiving dinner only to find the pea salad, the dinner rolls, and the cranberry sauce still in the refrigerator three days later.

...the timer goes off and you remove the pot roast from the oven after two hours, only to realize that you never turned the oven on.

...you are making a cake and have to start over dozens of times while measuring the dry ingredients because you keep forgetting how many cups of sugar and flour are already in the bowl.

While Cleaning and Doing Laundry...

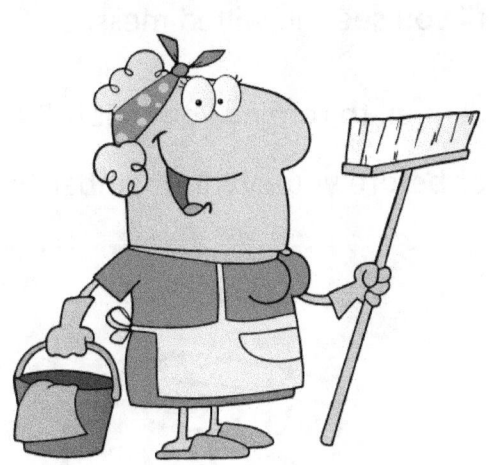

...you have a house cleaner come each week to help you maintain your studio apartment.

...your clothes rarely make it out of the laundry room to be folded because you keep forgetting that you washed them.

...you realize you have emptied the dishwasher and put the dirty glasses in the cupboard.

...you sweep the kitchen floor and empty the dustpan into the dishwasher.

...you add liquid potpourri to your mop water before realizing that it is not pine cleaner.

...you buy shredded lettuce for sandwiches but you put it in the freezer instead of the refrigerator, and have no recollection of doing it until you see the wilted mess.

...your husband sends you e-mail to remind you that he is out of socks and underwear before you ever remember to do laundry.

...the noise of the timers on the washer and dryer annoy you to the point you want to pull your hair out, but without them, the clothes sit in the washer for a month.

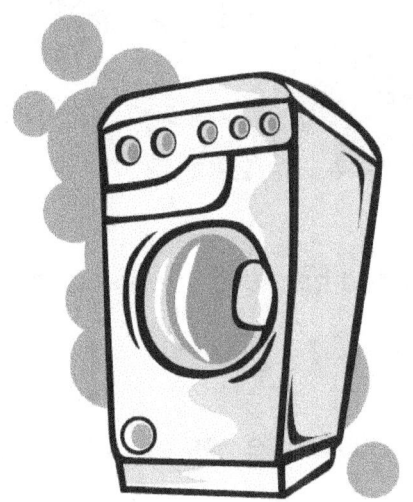

...your kindergartener has to wear your socks to school because you couldn't find her dirty socks.

...you find it easier to just go buy more socks and underwear than to find the ones you have.

...it takes you two days to clean a room that anyone else could clean in 15 minutes.

...cleaning cupboards, closets, and drawers in your house seems like Christmas because you find things that you don't even remember having in the first place.

...you find yourself searching the kitchen for that horrible smell and finally discover the pound of hamburger you defrosted in the microwave a week ago.

...when you finally do some cleaning, you find all the pens, scissors, super glue, and forks you thought your child took but really you hid them yourself.

...you have to rent a storage unit after running out of room in your garage for storing all of the supplies needed for all 40 hobbies you've taken up this year.

...you accidentally tossed the laundry in the trash because you used a trash bag to carry clothes out of the laundry room when you couldn't find any of the six laundry baskets.

...you turned on the washer to let it fill while gathering clothes from the bedroom, only to find out two hours later that you never put clothes in the washing machine.

...you realize you never turned on the dryer when you did laundry yesterday.

...you have been out of town for 3 days and when you come home you notice that you had left the iron on.

While Eating and Dining Out...

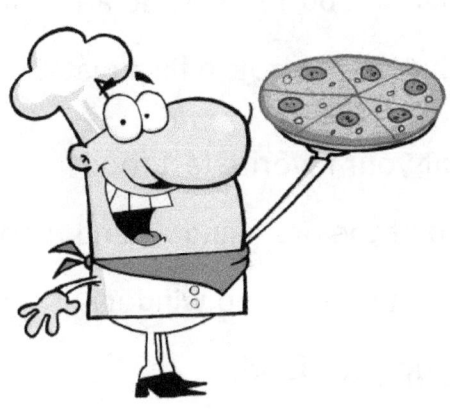

...people think you are a Vegan but its just that you keep forgetting to add meat to your recipes.

...your family asks you if you could be anorexic because you seem to be forgetting to eat.

...you order the same thing on the menu each time you visit your favorite restaurant because you are far too distracted to remember what you want before the server arrives to take your order.

...your friends insist on picking you up instead of meeting for lunch after the third time you went to the wrong restaurant.

...at least three times a week you get swallowing and inhaling confused and choke on your drink.

...you get all the way through the buffet line and arrive at your table only to realize that you forgot to fill a plate.

...you go to the drive thru at your favorite fast food restaurant, pay for the food at the first window and then hit the gas and drive right past the second window forgetting all about picking up your food.

...you leave a restaurant and two minutes later you have no clue what you had for lunch.

...you go to a seafood restaurant and ask for mild sauce.

...you go to serve green beans and find out you've cooked the lid too.

...you can drink coffee all hours of the day and into the night, and still fall asleep without a problem.

While Going to School or College...

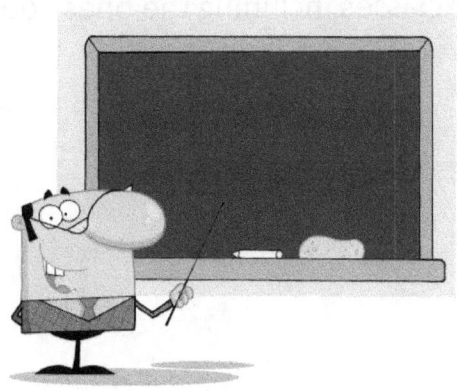

...you have been in college longer than the average doctor but still have no degree.

...you're listening to an instructor discussing an assignment. You cringe when he says, "I will only say this one time." You panic because you can't even remember it long enough to get it written down.

...you are given an assignment to write a book report but you write it about the wrong book.

...everyone in the class is given the same assignment but you interpret it completely different than anyone else in the room.

...you've spent three hours completing your homework only to forget to turn it in.

...you are failing all of your classes including the ones you have already taken before.

...it takes at least three tries to actually read one paragraph.

...you still spell like you talk.

...you have an entire notebook of rough drafts of your report after starting over after each mistake.

Your Friends and Family Know You Have ADHD When...

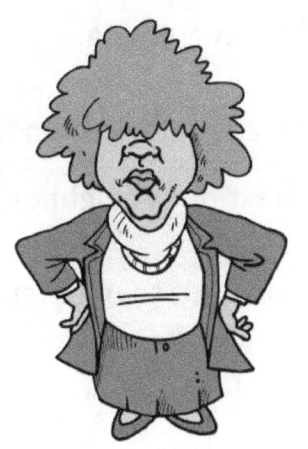

...you have difficulty following anyone's conversation.

...you constantly forget what you are saying in the middle of a sentence.

...you have to date five different people to get the perfect date.

...everything anyone says reminds you of a long story.

...you even interrupt a conversation when talking to yourself.

...you have been told that talking to you is like watching TV and you are controlling the remote.

...you feel that the only normal conversations you can have are the ones with others who have ADD.

...you lie awake in bed thinking of all the things you started to say to a friend but forgot until now.

...you have just celebrated your tenth anniversary but still don't have your name changed on everything.

...it has taken you months to realize that the friendly cashier at Walmart is also your next door neighbor.

...your friends and family find it difficult to understand your far reaching analogies.

...you start telling your husband an amazing discovery you made and he stops you by saying, "Dear, you've told me this story three times in the last 15 minutes."

...you just discovered a whole box of little gifts you intended to send to your daughter in college over a year ago.

...you forgot to be mad at your friend for something she did last week.

...everybody talks about how "amazing" and "incredible" you are, but then you say something real profound that makes them scratch their heads.

...your younger siblings remember your childhood better than you do.

...your neighbor downstairs reminds you each evening that you live up one floor.

...your friends can't understand you and tell you that you just need to learn time management.

...everyone around you thinks you've been really quiet lately but it's just because you are afraid to open your mouth for fear you will blurt out something really stupid.

...your friends are happy to trust you to keep their secrets because they know they will be erased from your memory permanently in the next five minutes.

...your family and friends take up a collection for an ADD evaluation and give you gift cards to cover the cost of the medication.

...you realize that the only thing worse than having ADD is living with someone else who has it.

...your kids re-wrap gifts for you from last Christmas and you don't notice.

...you visit that one friend who requires you to take off your shoes before you enter her home. When you arrive back at your house, you see that you are wearing two different shoes.

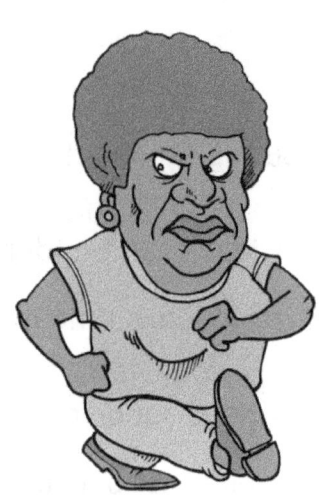

...your family is comprised mostly of ADD sufferers so family reunions are like a game of charades for the one who doesn't have ADD.

...you are talking with someone and they think you are purposely changing the subject when you have a dozen conversations in less than two minutes.

...your friends and family know better than to ask you what you were just thinking about.

...you wish people would talk faster so that you won't get distracted before they are finished.

...your friends laugh when you set an alarm to remind you to do something within the next 15 minutes.

...you lose something and your friends tell you to just retrace your steps. If you could possibly do that, the item would have never been lost in the first place.

...you explain your view on a situation and your friends say, "I've really never thought of it that way."

...your husband double checks his lunch when you pack it ever since you forgot the sandwich, drink and cookies and he had only an apple to eat.

...you think of a song every time someone talks because one line in the conversation matches a song you heard ages ago.

...you have lunch with the preacher's wife and about halfway through the meal you ask her what church she goes to.

...your friends give you blank stares when you blurt out the latest list of unrelated compelling thoughts that just ran through your mind.

...you see someone you haven't seen in ages and you run over and hug him, then hastily tell him the details of your adventurous life. He tells you that he has no idea who on Earth you are while he speeds away.

...you have several friends who say they would like to live closer to you just because your chaos is so entertaining.

...your friends tell you that it would be easier to communicate with you if they were on drugs.

...you have at least one friend who calls just to hear about your latest "ADD/ADHD moment."

Your Kids Know You Have ADHD When...

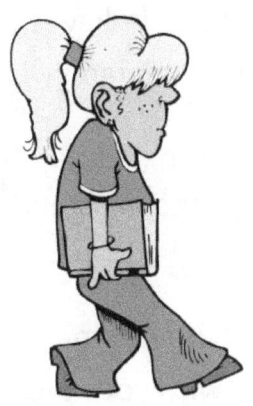

...you drop your child off at school and keep talking to her until you finally realize she's not even there.

...you take your infant son to the babysitter without a diaper.

...people who know you and know your kids unanimously agree that ADD is a genetic condition.

...your kids inform you that you have been lying about your age but not to appear younger.

...your daughter sends you a text to ask where you are. You tell her that you've just left the mall and she reminds you that she rode there with you.

...you work to convince your child that the tooth fairy is on vacation after forgetting to leave money under his pillow for a week.

...your daughter's boyfriend fears that you will reject him when you discover he has ADD but you welcome him to the family.

...your child's teacher tells you that she believes your child has ADD and you respond, "No, all of my family is like that."

...you work at the preschool that your son attends and still forget to pick him up.

...you can't help your third grader with her math homework because you still count with your fingers.

...you are well over 8-years-old but you still don't know your multiplication tables and you use your fingers to add.

...you and your labor coach have ADD so your first born son ends up being born in a convenience store parking lot after getting lost on the way to the hospital.

Your Idea of the Latest Fashion Means...

...your purse needs wheels after you pack it with stuff you never want to forget.

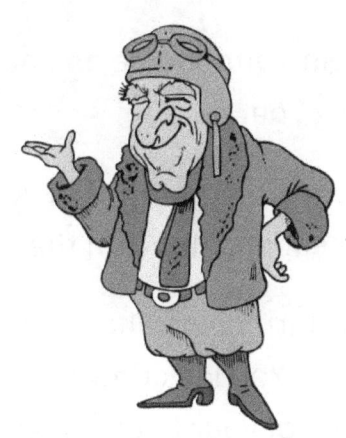

...you've lost your purse for the third time so now you cram all of your cosmetics into the pockets of your cargo pants.

...you realize you've worn your fluorescent purple bra under your white blouse to church.

...you have three holes pierced in each ear but never remember to wear earrings.

...you donate clothes to the thrift store and then accidentally buy them back.

...you have a small purse that is packed with everything you consider essential. You then decide to get a bigger purse, but suddenly it dawns on you that the size of the purse is not the problem.

...your spouse sets out clothes for work the night before and you wake up early and hang them up while he's in the shower.

...you put your hoodie on backwards and the hood is covering your face.

...someone points out that you are wearing three earrings on one ear and none on the other.

...you return home and see a strange set of footprints in the snow. You look down at your feet and see that you have one of your boots on and one of your husband's.

...you find a box of clothes you've intended to donate to the thrift store a year ago. Now you decide to start wearing them again.

While Managing Finances...

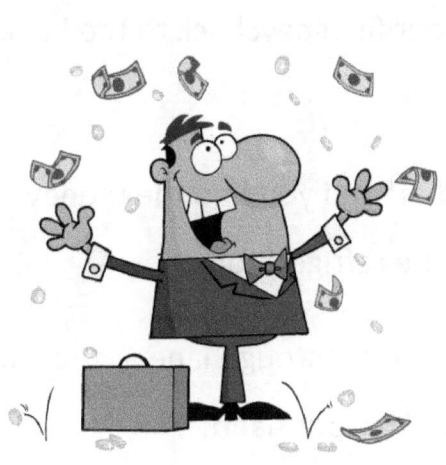

...you've left your debit card in the ATM machine more than twice this month.

...you have to file bankruptcy after your late fees total more than the credit card balance, even though you had the money to pay the monthly balance from the start.

...your new credit card arrives in the mail and you shred it thinking it was the old one.

...you lose your debit card when attempting to put it in the receipt slot at the gas pump.

...you have decided it is best that you don't own any credit cards so that you can avoid all of the impulsive purchases.

...you can't remember the answers to your security questions for online banking and you entered them.

...you still haven't taken your final paycheck to the bank after almost a year.

...your electricity is turned off and you find the money order under a magnet on the refrigerator.

...you attempt to leave the drive through lane at the bank with the money canister still in your hand.

...you have never sent in a rebate because you have never had the receipt, UPC code, and the rebate form in the same place.

...you consider duplicate checks one of greatest inventions of all time. Without those, your overdraft fees would be more than the mortgage.

...you never send in your monthly payments with the envelopes provided with your statements.

...you send your tax return by media mail because your stack of W-2s is as thick as a book.

...you order a burger from the dollar menu and your debit card is declined.

...you have not balanced your checkbook since 1982.

...you have three bank accounts but because you continuously use the wrong debit card, you pay more in overdraft fees than you do for groceries.

...you never remember which side of the car the gas tank is on even though you've owned the vehicle for over five years.

...you drive off with the gas pump nozzle still in your gas tank.

...you have grocery store receipts from 1989 in your purse but you can't find your debit card.

...you keep trying to type your employee identification number at the ATM machine thinking it is your PIN number.

...you have to call the bank several times each week to have your password reset, because you just can't remember the answer to the security question you provided.

...you check the unclaimed property website and find that you have left money in three bank accounts and forgot to pick up two pay checks.

...you frequently discover your lost wallet in the washing machine.

...you've had to report credit cards stolen three times this month because you've left your purse somewhere but have no idea where.

...you find money that you lost several months ago, which you never even knew was missing.

...the check your parents gave you for your birthday last year is still in your wallet.

...you have 3 different check books started and get totally confused with all of the out of sequence checks listed in your online banking account.

While Managing Health...

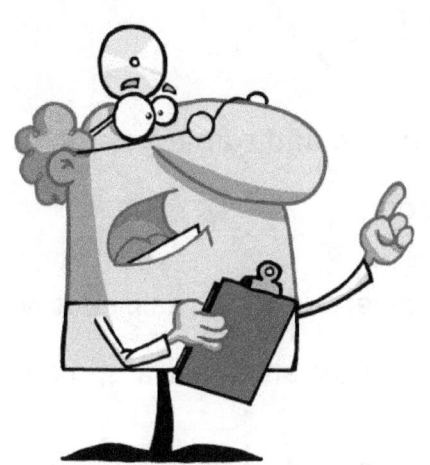

...you get infuriated when someone thinks ADD does not exist so you invite them to live with you for a week to make believers out of them.

...your spouse asks you how your day went and you sit there in a daze trying to remember just one thing you did all day.

...your friends say, "You don't have ADD. You just try to do too many things at once, won't sit still long enough to get anything done, and forget everything constantly!"

...you get upset when some alleged expert says, "ADD is a condition designed by the pharmaceutical industry." They obviously have never experienced the dynamics of ADD.

...you look like a victim of domestic violence with all of your bruises, but you have no idea how you got any of them.

...you are well over 2 years old and someone still reminds you to go use the bathroom.

...you started taking a shower but then realized it was dirty so you started cleaning the shower walls instead.

...you just got out of the shower and realize you've shaved one leg but forgot the other.

...you can't remember if you've already showered today or not.

...you are in the shower and you use the face scrub on your hair.

...you've overflowed the bathtub after you decided to wash the mop and then you became distracted and decided to cook supper instead.

...you are confused about whether you were getting in the bath tub or getting out.

...you start using 2-in-1 shampoo and conditioner so you won't have to remember which is which.

...you enter the bathroom and ask yourself, "Why am I here, again?"

...you are well stocked with toilet paper because you buy it every time you go to the store.

...you sit down to go to the bathroom and half an hour later you have completed an order form from a mail order catalog and can't figure out why your feet are asleep.

...you are flushing foot powder out of your eye.

...your family doctor tells you that you are too smart for ADD and way too young for Alzheimer's disease.

...you take a pill and two minutes later you have to count the pills to see if you actually did take it.

...your ADD medication lists suicidal thoughts as a side effect and you are concerned about forgetting that you had those thoughts.

...you upset the entire staff at the doctor's office when you suddenly decide to switch doctors and the new doctor is a partner of the former doctor.

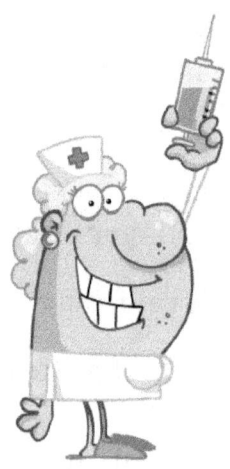

...people always think you are addicted to drugs but the only reason you act this way is because you are NOT taking any drugs.

...your pharmacy sends out a monthly reminder to let you know that you did not pick up your ADD medication.

...you go to the pharmacy to pick up a prescription but forget which child is the patient.

...you've sprained your ankle while just standing in the kitchen.

...you are depressed after taking your ADD medication when you realize that you actually kind of enjoyed being absentminded and disorganized!

...you are well over 40 and your mother still calls each day to remind you to take your medication.

...your husband put child locks on the medicine cabinet to keep you from accidentally taking his medication even when you forget your own.

...you decide you need to be officially diagnosed with ADD because your family has taken the self-test for you and diagnosed you as severely afflicted.

...people ask if you are feeling sick when you are caught up in a really deep daydream.

...you find yourself trying to curl your hair with your electric toothbrush.

...you find yourself daydreaming during meditation.

...your doctor asks you which ADD symptoms you are experiencing and you just can't remember even one of them.

...one of the primary reasons you are not an alcoholic is because you can't remember to stop at the liquor store.

...you realize you still have your glasses on when even after you've shampooed your hair.

...you are on the phone to poison control when you realize you just took your cat's medicine instead of your own.

...your face feels minty fresh after you used mouthwash on it instead of astringent.

...you carry a toothbrush and toothpaste with you in case you realize you've forgotten to brush your teeth before leaving the house.

...your reminder app beeps to let you know it is time to take your medication. You go to the medicine cabinet and can't remember what you came to get.

...you put a thermometer in your sick child's mouth and then start asking him questions.

...you go visit your doctor complaining of pain in your finger and she informs you that you had burned your finger sometime in the last month but you have no recollection of the injury at all.

...your doctor's nurse returns to the exam room to see why you are still sitting there when your visit was over 30 minutes ago.

While Trying to Sleep or Relax...

...your therapist suggests relaxation exercises but you have determined that they require too much concentration.

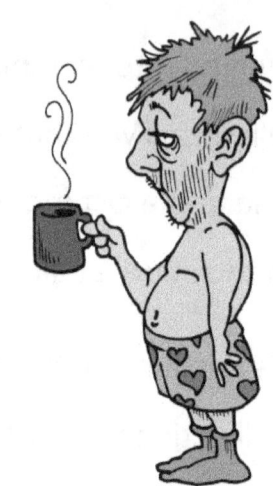

...you can sleep right through a tornado, but if water is dripping in the kitchen you can't fall asleep.

...you spend your whole day trying to stay alert and focused, then lie awake at night trying to get your brain to shut off.

...you sleep on top of your bed for days just to avoid having to make the bed every morning.

...you need to buy a new alarm clock every couple of months because your brain learns to tune out the sound of the alarm.

...you are suddenly awakened in the middle of the night with the most brilliant idea and by morning you've forgotten it.

...you keep a legal pad, a pen, and a book light by your bed. If you don't write down your important thoughts when they enter your head, in just seconds they will be gone forever.

...you've been sleeping on the floor for the past six months because it is too much work to clear off the bed.

...your spouse complains that the king size bed is not big enough and you realize that it is because your side is piled high with books, a laptop, a PDA and a legal pad.

...it seems like all the fun starts just ten minutes before you are supposed to go to bed.

While Getting Organized...

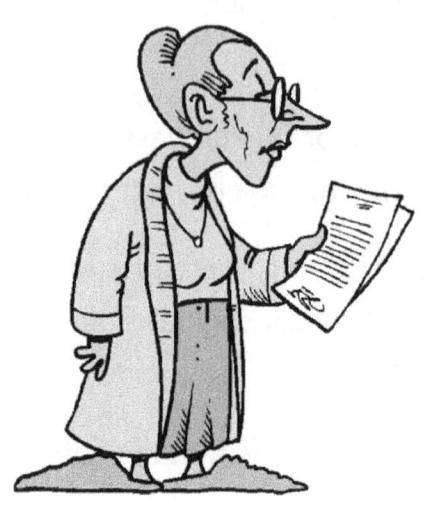

...your husband tells you that you are just one garage sale away from becoming a hoarder.

...you often drift off into daydreams of what life must be like for those who live an organized life without the stress of being late or forgetting anything.

...your to do list becomes your unfinished project list.

...you can't get anything done because you are too focused on what you have left to do.

...you over analyze everything to the point of being ridiculous.

...you realize that you can't remember something if you can't pay attention to it in the first place.

...you believe that everyone lives a life of total chaos, and absolutely won't accept that there are people that don't.

...you own an electronic organizer with alarms, a task manager, and a notepad but you aren't sure where it might be.

...you wonder how on Earth people without ADD can be so successful and have a relatively stress free life.

...you can be simultaneously logical, fervent, artistic, and methodical.

...doing the bizarre comes as second nature but it takes extraordinary achievement to do something normal.

...you make more messes than you have time to clean up.

...people are impressed to see the number of reminder and organization related apps on your iPhone.

...your idea of staying organized is having little yellow sticky notes on everything.

...people think you are kidding when you ask what year it is.

...you have a bookcase full of books that would help you get a handle on your disorganization but you are too distracted to read them.

...you forgot what you are looking for but keep looking because you are sure you will recognize it when you find it.

...you feel like you've spent half of your life trying to find something.

...you have a "safe place" for everything you don't want to lose but can't ever remember where that place might be when you need something.

Your Pet Knows You Have ADD When...

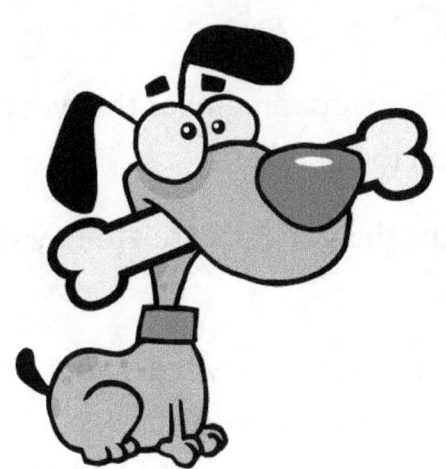

...you left your indoor dog outside all night.

...you know the whole family has ADD when you all return from the park and nobody knows where the dog is.

...you let your dog out in the back yard and remember he's there after you've been shopping in Walmart for an hour.

...you realize that the cat slept between the screen door and the front door all night because you didn't see her when you shut the door.

...your precious pets have discovered that if they drag their bowls to the middle of the kitchen, they have a better chance of getting fed.

...you constantly remind yourself not to forget the big bag of dog food on the bottom of the grocery cart before backing out of the parking space at Walmart.

...you miss the turtles and fish that you had as a kid but know that having them now would be far too cruel. You would forget to feed them.

...you arrive at the pet clinic only to remember that your cat is at home in his crate on the porch.

...you feel that the only living thing that can relate to you is your cat.

...you have forgotten the cat food so many times that your cat actually expects to have tuna every day.

...you and your dog are expelled from obedience classes because neither of you were paying attention in class.

...your cat follows you around the house meowing to remind you that you've forgotten to put fresh litter in the litter box that you cleaned two hours ago.

...you've found that your cat has leveled your house after you planted catnip in the living room.

...your cat knows your schedule better than you do and the only reason you get up is to get him off your chest.

...you complain to the police about the dogs barking next door. The officer then informs you that those neighbors don't have dogs and its actually your dogs barking so you will be getting a ticket for noise disturbance.

...your cat thinks you are trying to kill him when you pour bird seed in his dish and then leave for work.

...you have accidentally called your husband by your cat's name.

...you find something you lost in the bottom of the bag of dog food.

While Using a Phone...

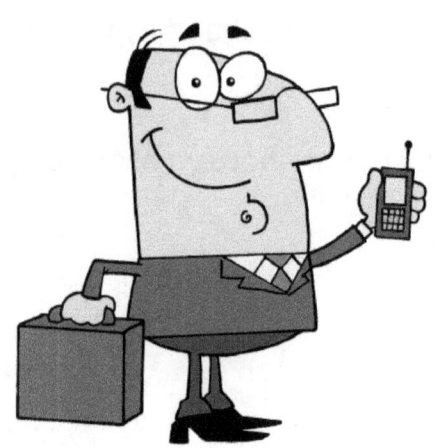

...you are so distracted by the music on hold that you forget which company you are calling.

...you send someone a text message but when they respond 60 seconds later, you've already forgotten what you asked them.

...you are desperately searching for your cell phone only to realize that you are talking on it.

...you leave your friend a 3-minute voice mail message consisting of a conversation you are having with your cat after you thought you hung up.

...you use your land line to call your mobile phone so you can find it and then you actually have to look and see who that "missed call" was.

...you use your land line to call your cell phone so you'll have the land line number.

...you are happy that there are now apps that let you use your phone as a remote for the TV.

...you keep getting distracted while talking to a friend on the phone and she has to ask more than ten times if you are still there.

...you forget who you are calling on the phone before the first ring.

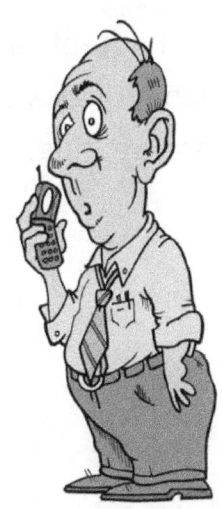

...your friends and family know to call you at least three times in a row on your cell phone because you won't find it the first two times.

...you are on the phone with your mom and are also chatting with tech support and balancing your checkbook at the same time.

...your friends think you screen your calls but three rings really doesn't allow you enough time to figure out whether the ringing sound is from under the couch or buried in a pile.

...you regret setting your cell phone on silent mode because now you can't call it with the other phone to find it.

...you have a special app on your cell phone to prevent you from accidentally calling your friends at 3:00AM while you are obsessed with cleaning up your contact list.

...you run around frantically looking for your cell phone and then when it rings, you discover it in the pocket of the hoddie you are wearing.

While Shopping...

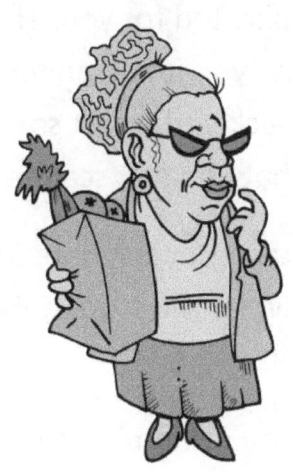

...you are near the top of the escalator when it suddenly stops. You call for help to get to the top.

...you went to the store to pick up one item and return home with five bags of groceries but forgot the item you went to get in the first place.

...you spent $200 at the grocery store and still have nothing to eat. The good news is that you have all of the salt, sugar, flour, and baking soda you'll need for a lifetime.

...the cashier rings up a bag of ice with your groceries but you always forget to pick it up on the way out.

...coffee was one of the items listed on your grocery list but you still forgot to put it in your cart.

...you have learned not to buy produce when going through self checkout at the grocery store. You forget the number on the apples three times before you can ever get it keyed in.

...self checkout is much too complicated for you. The voice tells you to put the item that you just scanned into the bagging area and you put it back in the cart so you have no idea which item it was that you just scanned.

...you live 10 miles from the nearest grocery store and at least three times a week you arrive at the store only to realize you don't have your wallet.

...you are halfway home before you remember that you paid for your groceries but left the cart inside the store.

...you try to make a grocery list but can't remember what you were going to write down before you went looking for a pen.

...you are frustrated because you can't get anything to come out of the vending machine but then you realize that you typed in the price and not the selection code three times.

While Driving or Traveling...

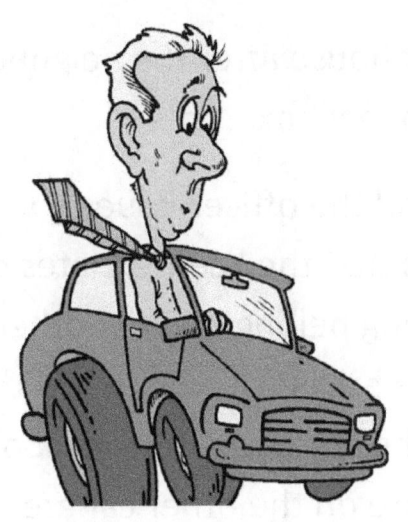

...you go to the kitchen to warm up your coffee only to realize that you've left your cup in the car.

...you get in your car, put it in reverse and are confused by that crashing noise until you see a tall tree in your rear view mirror.

...your husband yells, "We have made this trip seventeen times but on the eighteenth time, you manage to take a wrong turn. How does that work?"

...you are engrossed in a new book while riding the bus to work. You suddenly realize that you have missed your stop and have to get off the bus, cross the street and get on the bus going the other way.

You are thirty minutes late for work because you missed your stop again while reading the book.

...you couldn't find your house after the neighbors took down their custom mailbox.

...you are pulled over and the officer issues you a ticket after he discovers that the license plates on the vehicle you are driving belong on your other car. In a moment of true brilliance, you reveal that you must have gotten the stickers mixed up too because the ones that are on the other car are expired.

...you are pulled over and just as the police officer approaches your window, your five-year-old in the back seat says, "Hi Bill! I remember you. Is this a school zone too?"

...you have multiple copies of your driver's license after losing one and finding it later.

...police come knocking on the door to inform you that you left your car in neutral and it rolled into the neighbor's house.

...you consistently make the car behind you furious because you keep stopping at green lights.

...while driving you arrive at your final destination but can't remember why you are there.

...you missed that exit on the freeway and twenty minutes later you realized that you were not even close to where you were supposed to be.

...your spouse insists on living on a city bus route after you've forgotten to pick him/her up from work three times.

...you spend at least an hour wandering the Walmart parking lot looking for your car each time you shop.

...you use your cell phone to take a picture so that you'll remember where you parked your vehicle.

...you always wait until your low fuel warning light comes on before you stop to get gas.

...you make more than two trips around the block before you actually remember to turn into your own driveway.

...you drive down your own street and everything suddenly appears strangely unfamiliar.

...a parking garage makes you feel like you are trapped in a maze. You go past the exit three times before you ever get out to the street.

...you find construction zones very confusing because you can't ever figure out which side of the orange traffic cones you are supposed to be on.

...you start backing out of the driveway and can't remember for the life of you where you are going.

...your home is located at the foot of the Rocky Mountains but you still need a compass to figure out which way is West.

...you've confused a flashing light on a low bridge with a school zone and slowed down to 20 MPH.

...you never turn on your blinker until you are halfway around the corner because you cannot remember which way you are turning.

...you bring home more than three receipts from the same grocery store after each shopping trip.

...you fail the open-book driving test in front of your teen drivers.

...you never pay cash at a gas station because you go in to pay and drive off without pumping gas.

...you keep turning up the volume knob on the car stereo and then wonder why you still don't have cool air.

...your house comes into view and you see your other car in the driveway and wonder who is visiting.

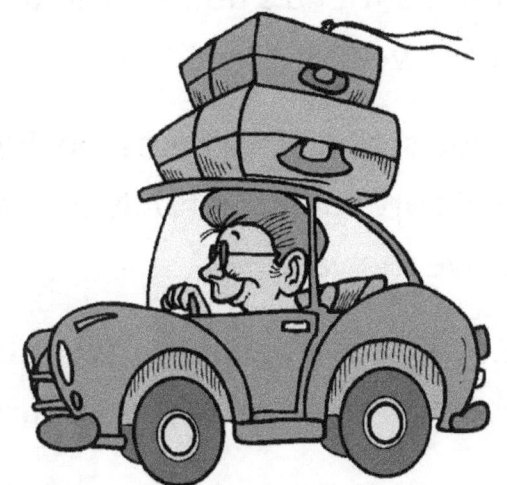

...you have four empty coffee cups and three empty fast food soda cups in your car.

...you could survive a natural disaster with just the items found in your car.

...you put your keys in your purse and leave it in the locked car.

...you won't use a GPS device because the audible driving instructions are too distracting.

...your GPS has recalculated your directions for the fourth time and now it tells you to turn around when possible.

...it takes you over a year to remember how to a get to a friend's house even when you go there every week.

...you spend 30 minutes looking for your car in the Walmart parking lot only to remember that you drove the van.

...every passenger who ever rides with you tells you how to drive, where to turn and when to stop.

...you put the trash in the trunk to take to the dumpster then wonder what in the world that horrible smell is in the car.

...the back seat of your car resembles a car owned by a hoarder.

...you are on vacation and the hotel clerk asks for your license plate number. You can't remember it to save your life even though it is a custom plate with your last name on it.

...your mechanic recommends that you drive a car with an automatic transmission after you have your transmission rebuilt twice from repeatedly starting out in second gear.

...your last vacation was over six months ago and your suitcase has still not been unpacked.

...the airlines insist on charging you to check your purse because it is too big to fit in the overhead compartment or under the seat in front of you.

...you finally find your car at the airport just seconds before you were ready to report it as stolen.

...you feel like you can relate to Moses wandering the desert for 40 years.

...you went to the wrong airport to pick up your visiting relatives.

...you leave the airport without remembering to go to baggage claim.

...you realize that some of your favorite travel destinations were discovered while you were lost.

...you are at the beach when it starts to rain so you pack up your stuff and leave. You get 25 miles down the highway and remember that you forgot your sisters who were in the restroom.

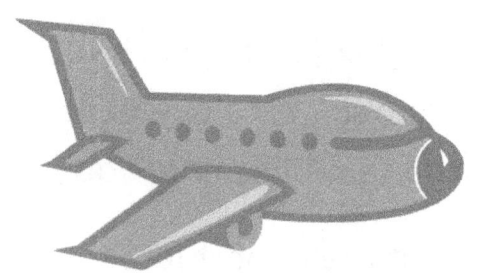

...your plane lands and as soon as you are in the terminal, you look at your boarding pass to see which city you are in.

...you and your sister are on a road trip and she sees an exit coming up and asks you to stop so she can use the restroom. You forget in the next few seconds and pass the exit. Now she's mad because it is ten miles until the next exit and insists that you pull over and let her drive.

...you stop to help someone with a car problem and lock your keys in your own car.

...you've attempted to replace the defective starter on your car but then realized you've put the old one back on.

...you realize that you are still repeating, "don't take the wrong turn" and you have no idea where you are.

...you go up and down each isle in the Walmart parking lot pressing the lock button on your car hoping you'll hear it so you can find it.

...you go right into panic mode when you get in your car and hear a voice screaming Swahili at you from the back seat. Then you find out the GPS unit was bouncing around in your purse and the language and volume level was changed.

...you come out of the office and realize you have not only left your keys in the ignition but the car is still running.

...you have to return to your home three times in the same morning to get something you forgot.

...your battery in your car's remote died just after you've bought groceries and you can't load the groceries into the car. You called your daughter to bring you the spare remote. She informs you that you can just use the key to open the car door and drive home.

While Working...

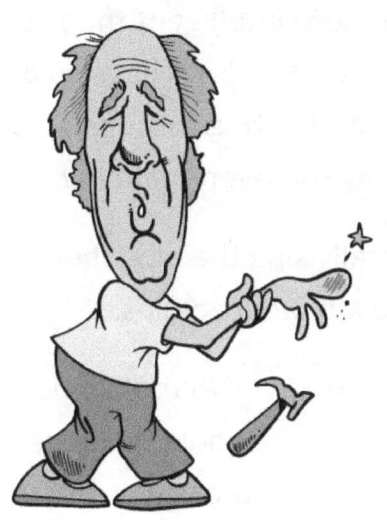

...it is impossible for you to take a half day of vacation. You always get distracted and take the whole day.

...you are always the last one to arrive at work in the morning and the last to leave at night.

...you're always way too busy, always on the go, and still never seem to get anything accomplished.

...your company buys pens in bulk and yet you can never find one when you need it.

...you regularly have the most astounding insights, but to the rest of the world they are considered blatantly obvious.

...you set your alarm for 5AM do you can be at work by 9:00AM and you are still late.

...you can't sit through a meeting, class, seminar or even church without doodling.

...you know you are much more intelligent than your boss with a master's degree is, but you don't have a college degree because the thought of sitting through all of those classes for a semester is way too overwhelming.

...you always have to mentally sing the alphabet song to yourself when you have to alphabetize files.

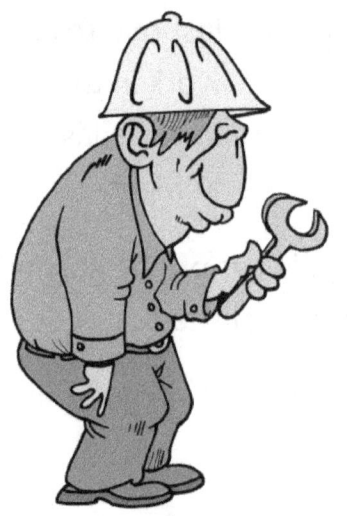

...your attention span would be longer if there weren't so many distractions around you.

...your friends and family admire your amazing ability to live "by faith alone" each day of your life.

...you are still trying to learn appropriate social behavior at the age of 45.

...you've been told that you can't accomplish anything because you are just lazy.

...you are known to be easily amused and quite entertaining but don't know why.

...telling you to pay attention and stay on task is like telling a blind man to just concentrate and he will see.

...someone suggests that you try meditation but you can't because you don't have a "quiet place" inside your head to go to.

...while taking an online ADD test, a pop-up ad for culinary school makes you hungry. Without blinking, you get up and go to the grocery store.

...you carry a small notebook with you so you can write down important thoughts before they fade from your mind.

...you arrive at the office and realize that your shoes don't match.

...you show up for work on your day off three weeks in a row.

...trying to listen to and follow instructions makes you feel very frustrated.

...you are halfway to work when you remember that you forgot to use deodorant.

...your kids think every day is "take your daughter to work day" because you keep forgetting to drop her off at her school.

...you wonder if ADD qualifies under the Americans with Disabilities Act for "reasonable accommodations" because you are too distracted by the quiet atmosphere and would like to get a TV and a radio in your office.

...you find that working for a temporary agency is right for you because you are likely to switch jobs every 30 days anyway.

...you have to have more than two sheets of paper to list all of the jobs you have had in the last five years.

...the lady from the payroll department constantly has to change your time sheet because you've tried to clock in twice but never clocked out.

...your resume is several pages long but there is no identifiable career path.

...you have been fired from your waitress job because you forgot the silverware, forgot the drinks and delivered the wrong meals to all of your customers.

...when something goes wrong at work, everyone points their fingers at you.

...you have arrived at work and just found out that you forgot to put a shirt on.

...your employer started charging you each time you lose your entry card or key fob.

...someone calls to leave a very important message for your boss but by the time you get off the phone you have already forgotten who called and what the message was.

...you absolutely cringe when people walk around the corner and seem shocked to see the size of the piles of paper on your desk.

...you are able to comprehend many instructions at once, but can't recall them later because they never had time to sink in before the next series of thoughts rushed in.

...you call in sick but your boss reminds you that you are already on vacation.

...you go to a job interview and your potential employer already has concerns about your ability to stay on task.

www.ingramcontent.com/pod-product-compliance
Lightning Source LLC
Chambersburg PA
CBHW071614170526
45166CB00003B/1079